MW01234628

In case of loss, please return to (+ as a reward):

_____

_____

_____

The 365 Journal For Men

One Year, Daily Writing Prompts

"Dwell on the beauty of life. Watch the stars, and see yourself running with them."

Marcus Aurelius

WEEKLY INSPIRATION 1

Date: 1 / 31 / 21

"I gaze forward without fear."

Alexander Pushkin

What qualities do you need to develop in order to reach your most important life goals?

① Discipline. Healthy eating has been a step in the right direction. It shows me that I have a level of resolve and am capable of change.

② Mindfulness. I have dabbled with "Untethered Soul" for years and have had hours and even days of mindfulness but have always reverted back to numbing out on meaningless distractions like sports, poker, video games, or television. Mindfulness will help me to unlock my purpose and develop life goals.

③ Creativity — I limit myself and put myself in a very narrow and confined box. Most things I think of as things "other people" do and not me I don't dream and I always focus on the negative or the obstacles. I need to get creative and explore everything that I may or may not be capable of. I need to try.

"I've started many times.. 2021 is going to be definitive in some way. I'm thankful for the past but I die today.. I am an ~~open~~ empty vessel. A blank canvas"
    —Brad

Date: 2 / 1 / 21

Write down the three most important lessons you learned in recent years.

① You can't fake wisdom and can never truly understand what someone is going through. Life changes and shapes us and its not always for the better. Take a step back and look inside on occasion. Give grace to everyone because they are likely trying their best and don't mean to be the twisted version of themselves.

② Perception is everything. We always have the ability to choose how we view something.

③ Don't give your mind away. It is getting easier and easier to do with technology. Some people numb out and give away their whole lives.

"Erase your personal narrative. It's mostly bullshit. Live"
-Brad

6

Date: 2 / 2 / 21

What does money symbolize in your life?

I honestly don't know. When I think of money I often associate it with student loan debt. Once we paid it off it has been a bit of a different feeling. I've often heard that money = options. I think that there is truth in that. For me, money has often equated to complacency. My wants and needs have always been fairly simple and if I can do basic things like go out to eat or place a few bets without having to worry about it, I don't feel compelled to pursue more. Since our house search has become more intentional, I do find joy in seeing the savings account for our house continue to climb. I'm glad that I don't obsess about money but in some ways I wish I cared more. I have achieved a level of success and decent earnings by some standards but am not sure if making more money would raise my self esteem. I need to spend more time on this question.

When was the last time your mind stopped your enthusiasm?
How did you feel about that?

My mind stops my enthusiasm a lot. I typically focus on the roadblocks and negatives. I just had a good meeting with co-workers but always worry, obsess and doubt after that I'll get in trouble.

Make a chronological list with the moments that made who you are today
when it comes to your love life/dating life.

Tina Hermanet
Nicole Guastella
Marisa Sciorrino
~~Dan~~ Ideene Dehclashti
Jo Farnum
~~Maggie Jaraucci~~
Mary Sweet
Isabel Abela
Katie Fazio
Kaitlyn Yutrepski — Janine Lizotte
Nicki Intalin
Liz Sherman
Genie Jacobs
Angie Depoto
Genna Buffa
Kelly Steiner
Megan Young
Mo
Bekdar Battler
Hilary Hutchins
Liz Bove
Nicole Callahen
Julie Przymusinihi

WEEKLY INSPIRATION 2

Date: 2 / 5 / 21

"For the person who has learned to let go and let be,
nothing can ever get in the way again."

Meister Eckhart

How would you describe masculinity?

Handling business is the first thing that comes to mind. Whether that be with physical strength or vulnerability. True ~~masculi~~ masculinity requires self awareness and emotional intelligence. I think the physical aspect does come into play as far as making food and fitness choices to help you be at your best both physically and mentally if called upon. Masculinity comes down to how we handle things.

What masculine qualities do you possess? What is the benefit of that?

How do mainstream media influence your view of the world?

Is your sexual energy enriching your life or is it enslaving you?
Explain your answer.

Write down the last time you told a lie to protect your image.

WEEKLY INSPIRATION 3

Date: /   /

"Re-examine all you have been told. Dismiss what insults your soul."

Walt Whitman

How has the relationship with your father determined who you are today?

_____

_____

_____

_____

_____

_____

_____

_____

_____

_____

_____

_____

_____

_____

_____

_____

_____

_____

_____

_____

_____

_____

Which emotion do you find most difficult to deal with and why?

_____
_____
_____
_____
_____
_____
_____
_____
_____
_____
_____
_____
_____
_____
_____
_____
_____
_____
_____
_____
_____
_____
_____
_____
_____
_____

Date: / /

Write down seven small things you can do to expand your comfort zone.

What uncertainties you once had, have now disappeared?

What does your *shadow-self* look like?

_____

_____

_____

_____

_____

_____

_____

_____

_____

_____

_____

_____

_____

_____

_____

_____

_____

_____

_____

_____

_____

_____

_____

_____

_____

_____

_____

_____

_____

WEEKLY INSPIRATION 4

Date: / /

"Happiness is like a butterfly which, when pursued, is always beyond our grasp, but, if you will sit down quietly, may alight upon you."

Nathaniel Hawthorne

Write down three things you can do this month to improve your career/business.

How would you describe femininity?

What feminine qualities do you possess? What is the benefit of that?

Date: / /

What role has advertising played in shaping your beliefs about men and women?

Date: / /

Why would people underestimate you?

WEEKLY INSPIRATION 5

"Let us not seek to satisfy our thirst for freedom by drinking from the cup of bitterness and hatred."

Martin Luther King Jr.

How has the relationship with your mother determined your love life/dating life?

_____

_____

_____

_____

_____

_____

_____

_____

_____

_____

_____

_____

_____

_____

_____

_____

_____

_____

_____

_____

Are your desires coming from your ego or your heart? Explain your answer.

Write down five things that make you an attractive romantic partner.

Write down five things you are seeking in a romantic partner.

If you could write the next chapter of your life right now, what would it look like?

_____
_____
_____
_____
_____
_____
_____
_____
_____
_____
_____
_____
_____
_____
_____
_____
_____
_____
_____
_____
_____
_____
_____
_____
_____
_____
_____
_____

WEEKLY INSPIRATION 6

Date: /   /

"The increasing seriousness of things, then that's the great opportunity of jokes."

Henry James

In what way is your dating life/love life a reflection of who you are?

_____

_____

_____

_____

_____

_____

_____

_____

_____

_____

_____

_____

_____

_____

_____

_____

_____

_____

Who was your role model while growing up?
What did you learn from him or her?

If you would meet your 21-year old self in a bar tonight, what is the one piece of advice you would give?

Do you sometimes feel superior to other people?
When and why?

Do you feel you often have to justify yourself to other people?
Why or why not?

Weekly Inspiration 7

"For there is a bigger you awaiting and the problems of today will soon be seen as small and insignificant tomorrow."

C.W. V. Straaten

Write down three things you can do this month
to improve your dating life/ love life.

_____

_____

_____

_____

_____

_____

_____

_____

_____

_____

_____

_____

_____

_____

_____

_____

_____

_____

_____

How do you most often seek approval in your life?

What would you miss if you stopped using your smartphone for 48 hours?

What kind of life do you think you deserve?
Is it far away from the life you are living now?

What kind of people do you look up to?
(Name at least three characteristics or behaviors)

WEEKLY INSPIRATION 8

Date: /   /

"The universe is wider than our views of it."
Henry David Thoreau

What masculine qualities would you like to develop more?

How is the way you treat your body going to affect you in 5 years?
And in 10 years?

Write down the three most common self-critical thoughts you have.
How can you deal better with these thoughts?

What are seven small things you truly enjoy?

Plan tomorrow exactly as you would want it to be,
and then try to follow it as closely as you can.

WEEKLY INSPIRATION 9

Date: /   /

"You only lose what you cling to."

Buddha

In what way is your health a reflection of who you are?

How has seeking approval affected your childhood?

Date: / /

How would you describe yourself?

Date: / /

How would the people closest to you describe you?

Date: / /

What leads your life, your intuition, or your mind?
Why?

_____

_____

_____

_____

_____

_____

_____

_____

_____

_____

_____

_____

_____

_____

_____

_____

_____

_____

_____

_____

_____

_____

_____

_____

_____

_____

_____

_____

_____

_____

_____

_____

WEEKLY INSPIRATION 10

Date: /   /

"Do anything, but let it produce joy."

Walt Whitman

What does sex symbolize in your life?

Date: / /

In what area of your life could you use some external help?

How has Hollywood/the movie industry affected
how you think a man 'should be'?

What is one new thing you would like to learn before you die?

What about your life would make other people jealous?

WEEKLY INSPIRATION 11

Date: /   /

"A very small degree of hope is sufficient to cause the birth of love."

Stendhal

Who would you like to be ten years from now?

What is your body trying to tell you over the past few months?

When and why are you being sarcastic?

Why do you have to improve yourself?

What dominating thoughts are running your life?

WEEKLY INSPIRATION 12

"What difference is there in the color of the soul?"
Solomon Northup

Imagine you met your 80-year old self tonight.
What would he or she tell you not to worry about?

What three things about the near future give you excitement?

What particular lesson is life trying to teach you?

Date: / /

What does integrity mean to you?

Where in your life are you not thinking for yourself?

WEEKLY INSPIRATION 13

Date: / /

"The most perfect life develops as a circle, and terminates in its beginning, making it impossible to say, This is the commencement, that the end."

Lew Wallace

What are your thoughts on the objectification of women/men and porn?

Date: / /

What song(s) reminds you of good times?

In what way(s) are you the same as your father?

In what way(s) are you different from your father?

What role does materialism play in your life?

Weekly Inspiration 14

Date: /   /

"There are no little things. Little things are the hinges of the universe."

Fanny Fern

Expressing yourself authentically is an attraction magnet.
How can authentic self-expression
help you to become more successful in life?

In your opinion, does the media share a message of hope and love, or of fear and negativity? What does this tell you about the media?

Date: /   /

In what way is your financial situation a reflection of who you are?

_____

_____

_____

_____

_____

_____

_____

_____

_____

_____

_____

_____

_____

_____

_____

_____

_____

_____

_____

_____

_____

_____

_____

What accomplishment from your childhood still brings a smile on your face? Why?

Date: / /

What three exciting things would you like to experience this year?

WEEKLY INSPIRATION 15

Date: /   /

"On a flimsy framework of reality, imagination spins, weaving new patterns."

August Strindberg

What blind spots have you detected in yourself over the last couple of years?

_____
_____
_____
_____
_____
_____
_____
_____
_____
_____
_____
_____
_____
_____
_____
_____
_____
_____
_____
_____
_____

Do you have a tendency towards narcissism or codependency?
How can you bring your relationships more in balance?

What is your opinion on multitasking?

Date: /   /

What would you like to change about the world?

_____
_____
_____
_____
_____
_____
_____
_____
_____
_____
_____
_____
_____
_____
_____
_____
_____
_____
_____
_____
_____
_____
_____
_____
_____
_____
_____
_____

Write down a long list of all the small actions you still need to do.

WEEKLY INSPIRATION 16

"A path is made by walking on it."

Zhuang Zhou

Write down the three most important lessons you learned
during your teenage years.

Date: / /

What is most often your first reaction in times of hardship?

How do you define taking care of yourself?

_____

_____

_____

_____

_____

_____

_____

_____

_____

_____

_____

_____

_____

_____

_____

_____

_____

_____

_____

_____

_____

_____

_____

_____

_____

_____

Look in the mirror for at least five minutes straight.
Reflect on what you saw and how you felt.

When was the last time you felt life was treating you unfairly?

Weekly Inspiration 17

Date: /   /

"You must be the best judge of your own happiness."

Jane Austen

Where are your thoughts?

If your thoughts are not 'in your head', what does this say about the 'I'?

Write down a memory, where you felt so worried,
but it all turned out to be okay.

_____
_____
_____
_____
_____
_____
_____
_____
_____
_____
_____
_____
_____
_____
_____
_____
_____
_____
_____
_____
_____
_____
_____
_____
_____
_____

When did someone surprise you, despite your doubts about him or her?

_____

_____

_____

_____

_____

_____

_____

_____

_____

_____

_____

_____

_____

_____

_____

_____

_____

_____

_____

_____

_____

_____

_____

_____

_____

_____

_____

Date: / /

Write down the last moment where you surprised yourself.

WEEKLY INSPIRATION 18

Date: / /

"Happiness originates from within.
Seeking it elsewhere is madness."

Zen Mirrors

Who and/or what do you believe is most in power on this planet?

Date: / /

In what way(s) can people only hurt you with your own consent?

Date: / /

Write down two or three accomplishments of recent years
that make you feel proud.

Write down two or three moments
that define where you are today when it comes to your career.

_____

_____

_____

_____

_____

_____

_____

_____

_____

_____

_____

_____

_____

_____

_____

_____

_____

_____

_____

_____

_____

_____

_____

_____

_____

_____

_____

Date: /   /

Do you believe in the statement
'You are always exactly at the right place, at the right time'?

Why or why not?

WEEKLY INSPIRATION 19

Date: /   /

*"Looking at these stars suddenly dwarfed my own troubles
and all the gravities of terrestrial life."*

H.G. Wells

What are your thoughts on extraterrestrial life?

When did you feel abandoned?

What can you say to that version of you who felt abandoned?

_____
_____
_____
_____
_____
_____
_____
_____
_____
_____
_____
_____
_____
_____
_____
_____
_____
_____
_____
_____
_____
_____
_____
_____
_____
_____

Write down three recent memories
when you felt you were helpful to other people.

What envy you once felt, is now gone?

_____

Weekly Inspiration 20

Date: /   /

"The imagination is not a state: it is the human existence itself."

William Blake

Have you ever done research on how the algorithms of your favorite social media companies (might) work? Why or why not?

_____

_____

_____

_____

_____

_____

_____

_____

_____

_____

_____

_____

_____

_____

_____

_____

_____

_____

_____

_____

_____

Have you ever done research on how Google algorithms (might) work?
Why or why not?

Write down one or two things you do that almost always bring you
in a state of negativity.

In what way(s) are all extremists
(left/right, religious/non-religious, etc.) the same?

Date: / /

What are your thoughts on racism?

Weekly Inspiration 21

Date: / /

"Above all else, never think you're not good enough."

Anthony Trollope

Write down three things you can do this month to improve your health.

What is your most empowering habit?
What about it makes it so strong?

Love is the way. To whom would you like to say some encouraging words?
And what would you like to say?

_____

_____

_____

_____

_____

_____

_____

_____

_____

_____

_____

_____

_____

_____

_____

_____

_____

_____

_____

_____

_____

_____

_____

_____

_____

_____

Date: /   /

What is your Inner Voice Trying to tell you in the last few months?

What do you think the world will look like in five years?

_____
_____
_____
_____
_____
_____
_____
_____
_____
_____
_____
_____
_____
_____
_____
_____
_____
_____
_____
_____
_____
_____
_____
_____
_____
_____
_____
_____
_____
_____

WEEKLY INSPIRATION 22

Date: / /

"Everyone sees what you appear to be, few experience what you really are."
Niccolò Machiavelli

What decisions do you need to make
to become the next best version of you?

Date: / /

What are your thoughts on inequality between men and women?

What talents are you hiding from this world?

Write down two or three recent memories when you felt truly peaceful.

Date: / /

What are three things you could do to build a healthier
and more passionate sex life?

WEEKLY INSPIRATION 23

Date: /   /

"Vision is the art of seeing things invisible."

Jonathan Swift

Write down a list of maximum seven thoughts that you frequently have that only bring you stress and unhappiness.

See yesterday's answer: rephrase these thoughts in an empowering way.

Which institutions, media outlets are you following without questioning?

In what area in your life do you find it difficult to find balance?

How would you treat the planet if it was a conscious living being?

WEEKLY INSPIRATION 24

Date: /   /

"I have no special talents. I am only passionately curious."

Albert Einstein

Write down three things you once thought were absolutely true, but now don't believe anymore. What does this say about your beliefs?

What is the beginning and what is the end of The Universe?
Or doesn't it exist?

And if not, what does that say about *beginning* and *end*?

How is the image you project to the world, other than your Authentic Self?

What do other people need to know about you, to understand you better?

What book(s) had a big impact on you during your teenage years? Why?

WEEKLY INSPIRATION 25

"Gratitude is not only the greatest of virtues but the parent of all others."
Marcus Tullius Cicero

If you could share one message in a Tv-broadcast for one billion people,
what would it be and why?

_____

_____

_____

_____

_____

_____

_____

_____

_____

_____

_____

_____

_____

_____

_____

_____

_____

_____

_____

How have you grown as a person in the last few months?

Why would people overestimate you?

What past failure actually proved to be a blessing?

Write down three things that other people can learn from you.

WEEKLY INSPIRATION 26

Date: / /

"Look beneath the surface; let not the several quality of a thing nor its worth escape thee."

Marcus Aurelius

What social conditions do you disagree with?

How can you be more truthful to others?

Write down a list of seven thoughts that always makes you feel better.

Write down three memories where Life/God/a Higher Power
really helped you in a surprising way.

What does being happy mean to you?

WEEKLY INSPIRATION 27

Date: /   /

"If you look the right way, you can see that the whole world is a garden."

Frances Hodgson Burnett

What is the main reason you feel the need to go
on this journey of self-discovery?

_____
_____
_____
_____
_____
_____
_____
_____
_____
_____
_____
_____
_____
_____
_____
_____
_____
_____
_____

Who determines where you look?
Who determines how you perceive what you look at?

What are your thoughts on inequality between the rich and the poor?

Date: / /

Write down three small things you can do this week
to reduce your stress level.

_____

_____

_____

_____

_____

_____

_____

_____

_____

_____

_____

_____

_____

_____

_____

_____

_____

_____

_____

_____

_____

_____

_____

_____

_____

_____

_____

_____

_____

What would the 7-year old version of you, think about you today?

Weekly Inspiration 28

"There is nothing in the world so irresistibly contagious as laughter and good humor."

Charles Dickens

How you think the world sees you.

Date: / /

How do you think the world will look like in twenty years?

Make a chronological timeline with the most significant incidents
that define who you are today.

Date: / /

The best 7-day diet that would work for you.

When was the last time you were too hard on yourself?

WEEKLY INSPIRATION 29

Date: /   /

*"To be what we are, and to become what we are capable of becoming,
is the only end of life."*

Robert Louis Stevenson

When was the last time you did something impossible?

_____

_____

_____

_____

_____

_____

_____

_____

_____

_____

_____

_____

_____

_____

_____

_____

_____

_____

_____

_____

_____

_____

_____

What rules are standing in the way of your happiness right now?

Date: / /

What are your thoughts on the law of attraction?

How could you loosen up a bit more?

Date: /   /

Write down three things you can do this month
to improve your financial situation.

Weekly Inspiration 30

Date: /   /

"There is a pleasure in the pathless woods."

Lord Byron

What past experience still runs your life in a negative way?

Look at yesterday's answer.
Write down three ways to deal better with this.

Date: / /

What are your thoughts on social anxiety?

What frustrates you the most about your sex life?

_____
_____
_____
_____
_____
_____
_____
_____
_____
_____
_____
_____
_____
_____
_____
_____
_____
_____
_____
_____
_____
_____
_____
_____
_____
_____
_____
_____

Date: / /

How does your ideal morning routine look like?

Weekly Inspiration 31

Date: / /

"If we take care of the moments, the years will take care of themselves."
Maria Edgeworth

Write down your personal manifesto on how to live life.

_____

_____

_____

_____

_____

_____

_____

_____

_____

_____

_____

_____

_____

_____

_____

_____

_____

_____

_____

_____

Date: / /

What are you chasing in life?
How can you attract it into your life instead?

The truth is the potential for growth after making a mistake is huge.
Why then, are we so afraid of making mistakes?

What is the goal of humanity?

Date: / /

Write down three small things you can do next week
to improve your productivity.

WEEKLY INSPIRATION 32

"Only the hand that erases can write the true thing."

Meister Eckhart

Everything you see around you was once thought.
What does this tell you about the mind?

Date: /   /

Money is neutral. What good things can you do with money?

_____

_____

_____

_____

_____

_____

_____

_____

_____

_____

_____

_____

_____

_____

_____

_____

_____

_____

_____

_____

_____

_____

_____

_____

_____

_____

_____

What bad things can you do with money?

What beliefs about love you once had, are now gone?

How would you describe time?
What is the purpose and meaning of it?

WEEKLY INSPIRATION 33

Date: / /

"Never say you know the last word about any human heart."

Henry James

Write down three strategies you can use to give your business/career a boost in the coming months.

Date: / /

What does being successful mean to you?

Date: / /

What simple pleasures did you enjoy this week?

Write down five simple things you can do when you feel down.

Date: / /

Write down a long list of all the things that make you feel grateful
for your current situation.

_____

_____

_____

_____

_____

_____

_____

_____

_____

_____

_____

_____

_____

_____

_____

_____

_____

_____

_____

_____

_____

_____

_____

_____

_____

_____

WEEKLY INSPIRATION 34

Date: / /

"To reach something good, it is useful to have gone astray."

St. Teresa of Avila

Describe the characteristics of a good friend.

What conversations you had this year gave you new insights about life/yourself?

Is your social life a true reflection of who you actually are?
Why or why not?

What beauty did you see this year?

_____
_____
_____
_____
_____
_____
_____
_____
_____
_____
_____
_____
_____
_____
_____
_____
_____
_____
_____
_____
_____
_____
_____
_____
_____
_____

Write down three things you can do to improve the living conditions in your home.

WEEKLY INSPIRATION 35

Date: / /

"How many things have been denied one day,
only to become realities the next!"

Jules Verne

Write down three things you can do to improve your sleep.

Write down seven reasons why you love yourself.

Write down seven reasons why you love humanity.

Date: / /

Write down three things you can do to deal better with worries.

Date: / /

What act of kindness did you witness this week?

WEEKLY INSPIRATION 36

Date: /   /

"I believe that unarmed truth and unconditional love will have the final word in reality. This is why right, temporarily defeated, is stronger than evil triumphant."

Martin Luther King Jr.

Describe your ideal three weeks of traveling.

Date: / /

What do you have to give up to live a more authentic life?

Date: /   /

When was the last time you felt truly alive?

What new places in or around your hometown can you visit this year?

_____

_____

_____

_____

_____

_____

_____

_____

_____

_____

_____

_____

_____

_____

_____

_____

_____

_____

_____

_____

_____

_____

_____

_____

_____

_____

Describe your ideal workweek.

WEEKLY INSPIRATION 37

Date: / /

"When you are finished changing, you're finished."

Benjamin Franklin

Write down three things you can do this month to make your ideal travel plans come to fruition.

_____

_____

_____

_____

_____

_____

_____

_____

_____

_____

_____

_____

_____

_____

_____

_____

_____

_____

_____

_____

_____

_____

Write down one or two important turning points in your life.

How would you spend a million dollars?

Imagine you earned twice as much per month than you earn now: write down an exact budget of how you would spend that money.

What three things can you do to improve your relationship with yourself?

WEEKLY INSPIRATION 38

Date: / /

"If the rules are such that you can't make progress, then you have to fight the rules."

Elon Musk

What do you hide from most people?

Date: / /

What mistakes do you constantly repeat,
when it comes to your dating life/love life?

_____
_____
_____
_____
_____
_____
_____
_____
_____
_____
_____
_____
_____
_____
_____
_____
_____
_____
_____
_____
_____
_____
_____
_____
_____
_____
_____

See yesterday's answer: write down three things you can do
to transcend these 'mistakes'.

What do you think your country will look like in five years?

A list of material things that make you feel happy.

Weekly Inspiration 39

Date: / /

"Do not be anxious about tomorrow, for tomorrow will be anxious for itself. Let the day's own trouble be sufficient for the day. "

Jesus Christ

In what area of your life do you experience scarcity?

In what area of your life do you experience abundance?

How are you most frequently misunderstood by other people?

Make a timeline of how you would want your life
to turn out to be over the next 10 years.

What problems in your life could actually be opportunities?

WEEKLY INSPIRATION 40

"When I let go of what I am, I become what I might be."

Jesus Christ

Write down three things you can do this month to improve your charisma.

Five statements you wanna live by.

Date: / /

What do you appreciate about your friendships?

Describe your Inner Critic.
What would be an appropriate name for him/her?

Date: / /

How does fear show up in your life?

WEEKLY INSPIRATION 41

"All the darkness in the world cannot extinguish the light of a single candle."

St. Francis Of Assisi

Write down three things you can do this week to start your days better.

What needs you have, do you need to take care of soon?
How can you do this without exhausting yourself?

Date: /   /

How can you take (better) care of your best talent(s)?

What would you like to learn about dealing with conflict?

Date: / /

Three uncommon things you can do this month.

Weekly Inspiration 42

"There is no greatness where there is not simplicity,
goodness, and truth."

Leo Tolstoy

What one small thing can you do on a daily basis
that would improve your life massively?

Who would you like to be three months from now?

Date: / /

What habits bring you more bad than good?

What makes you different from other people?

_____
_____
_____
_____
_____
_____
_____
_____
_____
_____
_____
_____
_____
_____
_____
_____
_____
_____
_____
_____
_____
_____
_____
_____
_____
_____
_____
_____
_____

What makes you the same as other people?

Weekly Inspiration 43

Date: /   /

*"With an eye made quiet by the power of harmony,
and the deep power of joy, we see into the life of things."*

William Wordsworth

What was your first experience with success?

What was your first experience with failure?

Describe your comfort zone.

Why is the comfort zone so closely related to the mind as a whole?

Date: / /

Times where strangers helped you in unexpected ways.

Weekly Inspiration 43

Date: / /

*"With an eye made quiet by the power of harmony,
and the deep power of joy, we see into the life of things."*

William Wordsworth

What was your first experience with success?

What was your first experience with failure?

_____

_____

_____

_____

_____

_____

_____

_____

_____

_____

_____

_____

_____

_____

_____

_____

_____

_____

_____

_____

_____

_____

_____

_____

_____

_____

_____

_____

_____

_____

Date: /   /

Describe your comfort zone.

Why is the comfort zone so closely related to the mind as a whole?

Times where strangers helped you in unexpected ways.

WEEKLY INSPIRATION 44

Date: / /

"Believe nothing you hear, and only one half that you see."

Edgar Allan Poe

What small things can you do this week to improve yourself?

Write down a memory, where you did everything to be in total control,
but then it seemed you weren't in control after all.

Date: / /

Write down a long list of things that make you feel grateful
for your childhood.

227

What have others liked about you, that you didn't notice yourself?

What advice would you give to yourself one year ago?

Weekly Inspiration 45

Date: / /

"The rights of every man are diminished
when the rights of one man are threatened."

John F. Kennedy

How does your pattern of procrastination look like?

Describe your ideal date night.

What makes you an unattractive romantic partner (relationship/dates)?
How can you work on this?

How can you better deal with your own prejudices?

Write down five characteristics you value in others.

WEEKLY INSPIRATION 46

Date: / /

"The trouble is, you think you have time."

Buddha

What beliefs did you borrow from other people?

Believes you hold, that actually don't serve you any longer.

Date: / /

Activities you do often, that actually don't serve you any longer.

Date: / /

What people are you fascinated by and why?

Date: /   /

How can you take better care of yourself in moments of uncertainty?

WEEKLY INSPIRATION 47

"Your days are numbered. Use them to throw open the windows of your soul to the sun. If you do not, the sun will soon set, and you with it."

Marcus Aurelius

Write down three small things you can do this week
to work on your most important goals in life.

Write down three moments in your life you would like to relive.

What courageous choice you made as a teenager is still benefiting you today?

Date: / /

In what area of your life are you struggling the most and why?

In what area of your life are you most successful?
What lessons can you learn from that?

WEEKLY INSPIRATION 48

Date: / /

"Never give up... No one knows what's going to happen next."

L. Frank Baum

Reflect on the relationship you have with yourself.
What is good about it?

What can you do better?

_____

_____

_____

_____

_____

_____

_____

_____

_____

_____

_____

_____

_____

_____

_____

_____

_____

Date: / /

Describe your ideal night out with friends.

What advice would you give your teenage self about life?

_____

_____

_____

_____

_____

_____

_____

_____

_____

_____

_____

_____

_____

_____

_____

_____

_____

_____

_____

_____

_____

_____

_____

_____

_____

_____

Date: / /

Write down three reasons why you can be optimistic about humanity?

Date: / /

Write down three things you would love to do
when you wake up tomorrow.

WEEKLY INSPIRATION 49

*"To put everything in balance is good,
to put everything in harmony is better."*

Victor Hugo

Write down three simple things you can do to develop your sense of humor.

How can you become less stifled, less serious?

Date: / /

If you died today, what would you regret not doing?

_____

_____

_____

_____

_____

_____

_____

_____

_____

_____

_____

_____

_____

_____

_____

_____

_____

_____

_____

_____

_____

_____

_____

_____

_____

Write down a list of all the things you're fascinated by
when it comes to money.

_____

_____

_____

_____

_____

_____

_____

_____

_____

_____

_____

_____

_____

_____

_____

_____

_____

_____

_____

_____

_____

_____

_____

_____

Write down a list of all the things you're fascinated by
when it comes to your preferred sex.

WEEKLY INSPIRATION 50

Date: / /

*"When the Soul wants to experience something she throws out
an image in front of her and then steps into it."*

Meister Eckhart

If you were granted one wish of any kind, what would you wish for?

What reward(s) are you seeking in your life and why?

What would happen if you did everything the opposite of how you normally do things for the next 24 hours?

If you died today, what would you regret not saying?

Write down all the reasons why you deserve to live a happy
and successful life.

_____
_____
_____
_____
_____
_____
_____
_____
_____
_____
_____
_____
_____
_____
_____
_____
_____
_____
_____
_____
_____
_____
_____
_____
_____

WEEKLY INSPIRATION 51

"Stop trying to change the mirror. All that's brought to you is a mere reflection. It's life bouncing back. The thoughts. The being."

C.W. V. Straaten

If you died today, what would you regret not seeing?

Write down a list of all the things you're fascinated by
when it comes to physical appearance.

_____
_____
_____
_____
_____
_____
_____
_____
_____
_____
_____
_____
_____
_____
_____
_____
_____
_____
_____
_____
_____
_____
_____
_____
_____
_____
_____

If you could eliminate one thing from your life today, what would it be? Why?

Date: /   /

Write down your biggest limiting beliefs about yourself.

Date: /   /

Look at yesterday's answer. Write down at least one reason why these
limiting beliefs no longer have the power over you, they used to have.

WEEKLY INSPIRATION 52

"Who in the world am I? Ah, that's the great puzzle."

Lewis Carroll

What has made life worthwhile for you?

Date: /   /

Who are you becoming?

_____
_____
_____
_____
_____
_____
_____
_____
_____
_____
_____
_____
_____
_____
_____
_____
_____
_____
_____
_____
_____
_____
_____
_____
_____
_____
_____

What should be your next step in life?

What has life been trying to teach you over the past few months?

Date: /   /

Write down a letter to yourself, to be opened six months from now.

This has been:

The 365 Journal For Men

One Year, Daily Writing Prompts

Made in the USA
Monee, IL
28 January 2021

58937064R00163